I BEAT CANCER

HOLISTICALLY

I BEAT CANCER

HOLISTICALLY

Protocols for Breast, Colon, Lung and Prostate Cancer

DANIEL J. GOLDSTONE

Wasteland Press

www.wastelandpress.net
Shelbyville, KY USA

I Beat Cancer Holistically:
Protocols for Breast, Colon, Lung and Prostate Cancer
by Daniel J. Goldstone

First Printing – November 2012
ISBN: 978-1-60047-783-6

The author is not a medical doctor, and the material in this book is not intended to diagnose, treat, cure or prevent any disease or illness. The information is not FDA approved, and is designed for educational purposes only, and should not be taken as medical advice or used as a substitute for medical care. Always consult with your health care provider before making changes in your diet, exercise regimen, or taking supplements or other natural remedies.

Use of any information contained in this book is at the sole discretion and risk of the reader. The author is not responsible for any adverse effects or consequences that may result, either directly or indirectly, from following the protocols contained herein, and makes no guarantees on the outcome of recovery.

Edited by Brenda Judy, www.publishersplanet.com

Printed in the U.S.A.

0   1   2   3   4   5   6   7   8   9   10

In loving memory of my father,
Harold S. Goldstone

Table of Contents

Acknowledgments

A special thank you to my mother, Rita M. Goldstone, and my sister, Sherri Joseff, for their help, input and support.

Introduction

You are probably wondering how you got cancer. No one can give you a definite answer, but it is probably a combination of factors: lifestyle, diet, genetics and environment. I learned a long time ago, you get out the same way you got in. You need to change your diet, lifestyle and actually improve your environment. As far as genetics, some supplements have actually been able to turn off the switch of defective genes.

Do you realize that you are responsible for the cause of this disease? The medical community totally ignores this critical point. The way they treat cancer is cut, burn and poison. These only deal with the symptoms. Why don't we deal with the cause? The result of traditional treatment is a weakened immune system, which causes a buildup of your free radicals. That is why our cancer treatments results are awful. Now, I am not saying I'm against traditional cancer treatment, what I am against is that it totally ignores the cause.

I am writing this book in order to help extend and save lives. My prior book, *Advanced Prostate Cancer and Me*, has helped people all over the world, from Cairo, Egypt, to Montreal, Canada. My approach has evolved over a seven-year period, and it is based on my science research as well as what others have conveyed to me with questions and experience. I am also doing what needs to be done. There are diet books about cancer, but not one that encompasses diet, supplements, lifestyle, mind, and how to use your mind, body and spirit to defeat the beast. I am not a big fan of books regarding your pH. They ignore your mind and soul. Again, not addressing 70 percent of the equation. We are not just a body; we have a mind, which is very powerful. We have a soul, which lives beyond our body.

Finally, I want to address why, if I had advanced prostate cancer, do I have protocols for breast, colon and lung cancer? First, all cancer is caused by the same thing, a weakened immune system. Second, breast cancer is caused genetically by the BRCA2 gene in both males and females, with the male getting prostate cancer and the female breast cancer. They are both a sex hormone cancer. Since my main five ingredients work on all four cancers, I learned that with minor modifications my approach should be effective for prostate, breast, lung and colon cancers. I firmly believe that my five main ingredients should work on most other cancers as well. It can also slow down the aging process, too.

I truly believe that it wasn't luck that I found these fantastic supplements; I had God working through me and others for me. I also believe it is my destiny to help people beat this beast, and I hope and pray that this approach saves and extends many lives.

Chapter One
My Story

In May 2005, I received the shock of my life when I was diagnosed with advanced cancer. My biopsy couldn't have been worse; all twelve samples showed cancer cells up to 75 percent. In addition, the cancer had escaped the prostate gland, and was in the surrounding tissue and nerves, which classified me as stage 3 cancer. It also could have been in other parts of my body—the scans only pick up masses of cells in the billions, not individual cancer cells.

After receiving the biopsy report from my doctor along with his recommended treatment, I decided to consult with other cancer specialists. After meeting with a couple of them, I started to get quite depressed. All of their treatment options would put an end to my sex life and potentially leave me with absolutely no feeling in my penis. At the time, I was fifty-three, single and not dating anyone. How could I expect any woman to share a life with an impotent man? To me, this meant I would die alone.

Desperate to find something that would effectively deal with the cancer and save my sex life, I started researching the Internet for a holistic approach to my situation. By mid-June, I was taking two different remedies and determined not to have any traditional treatment when one doctor finally recommended a treatment that would be the most effective with the least disruption to my lifestyle. After talking to all the doctors, researching the Internet and waiting almost two months since being diagnosed, I chose six months of hormone treatment (two LHRH hormone shots, each lasting three months), waiting two months after the first hormone shot, then doing thirty-nine external beam radiation treatments.

```
                Chart Review Copy - Duplicate Printout
           Requested by:  Croxton,Denise at:  05/23/05 1412
                William Beaumont Hospital - Royal Oak
                RO Surgical Pathology Report (Tamtron)

Patient Name  DOB:01/04/1952  Patient No   FC  Patient No  Dictation Date
Goldstone,Daniel J              1051745-05   30      SP       17 May 05  000

                                                        Page  1 of 2
```

```
   Case #   ROS-05-26591

   SPECIMEN: A. PROSTATE BIOPSY, LEFT; B. PROSTATE BIOPSY, RIGHT
   PRE-OP DIAGNOSIS:
   POST-OP DIAGNOSIS:
   CLINICAL INFORMATION:    Elevated PSA


   MICROSCOPIC DIAGNOSIS:
   * * * * * * * * * * * * * * * * * * * * * * * * * * * * * * * *
     * * POSITIVE RESULT * * POSITIVE RESULT * * POSITIVE RESULT * *
   * * * * * * * * * * * * * * * * * * * * * * * * * * * * * * * *


   A. PROSTATE, LEFT, BIOPSY
   --- ADENOCARCINOMA, GLEASON SCORE 7 (3+4)
   --- ADENOCARCINOMA INVOLVES 50% OF ONE NEEDLE CORE
   --- ADENOCARCINOMA INVOLVES 50% OF SECOND NEEDLE CORE
   --- ADENOCARCINOMA INVOLVES 75% OF THIRD NEEDLE CORE
   --- ADENOCARCINOMA INVOLVES 50% OF FOURTH NEEDLE CORE
   --- ADENOCARCINOMA INVOLVES 75% OF FIFTH NEEDLE CORE
   --- ADENOCARCINOMA INVOLVES 50% OF SIXTH NEEDLE CORE

   B. PROSTATE, RIGHT, BIOPSY
   --- ADENOCARCINOMA, GLEASON SCORE 7 (3+4)
   --- ADENOCARCINOMA INVOLVES 33% OF ONE NEEDLE CORE
   --- ADENOCARCINOMA INVOLVES 10% OF SECOND NEEDLE CORE
   --- ADENOCARCINOMA INVOLVES 5% OF THIRD NEEDLE CORE
   --- ADENOCARCINOMA INVOLVES 33% OF FOURTH NEEDLE CORE
   --- ADENOCARCINOMA INVOLVES 25% OF FIFTH NEEDLE CORE
   --- ADENOCARCINOMA INVOLVES 5% OF SIXTH NEEDLE CORE

   GROSS:

   A.  Received in formalin labeled "left prostate biopsy" are six needle
   cores of tan-yellow soft tissue ranging from 1.8 to 2 cm. Multiple/2, no G.

   B.  Received in formalin labeled "right prostate biopsy" are six needle
   cores of tan-yellow soft tissue ranging from 1.7 to 1.8 cm. Multiple/2, no
   G. mjd/nsg a

   Special procedures: Step sections A and B

   POSITIVE BIOPSY

                              Name of Report   Complete
                              RO Surgical Pathology Report
                              (Tamtron)
```

To make a long story very short, my treatment was much worse than the cancer. The usual and unusual side effects of their treatment were a living hell. Some of the side effects from the initial chemical castration were vertigo, insomnia, constant urination, massive headaches, no energy, depression, loss of muscle mass and impotence.

I lived that way for six months. It was the worst six months of my life. Now I know what hell is like. The only way I was able to cope with it was to keep telling myself it was only temporary; otherwise, I would have killed myself.

Nevertheless, about a week after I started the first hormone treatment, I consulted with a holistic doctor. After testing my blood for things I didn't know existed, he prescribed a list of supplements. Approximately two weeks later, I awoke one morning feeling different. It felt as though my prostate had shrunk and the cancer was going away (this was before the side effects of the hormone shot kicked in and before my radiation treatments). My beliefs were confirmed with a blood test. Week after week, my PSA continued to drop on the average of 40 percent, but the holistic approach did not stop the unbearable symptoms of the traditional treatments.

Disgusted with the side effects of the hormone shots and radiation, I wanted to stop them and just continue with the holistic approach. However, even though my doctor said I was doing well above average, he did not believe the supplements were the reason for my progress, and convinced me to continue with traditional treatment.

After enduring the worst six months of my life, my cancer returned nine months later with a vengeance. It was growing at 300 percent a month. My doctor suggested that I be chemically castrated to slow down the cancer. I may have considered that, however, I had just met my girlfriend, who was twenty-one years younger, and I wanted to enjoy the time we spent together. Therefore, I respectfully refused his recommendation and requested he retest me in thirty days.

At the time, I didn't know what to do. However, whatever I decided upon, I needed to do fast. The first thing I decided to do was modify my holistic approach. One day, while my girlfriend and I were at the health food store, she came across a supplement that was supposed to put certain cancer cells in a suspended state. I immediately added that along with tart cherry juice to my supplement regimen.

On August 18, 2006, my PSA dropped slightly to 2.17, but I was still not out of the woods because my PSA needed to be less than 1.0. On October 11, 2006, my PSA dropped to 1.82. It was still not low enough but I thought as long as I had a negative velocity, my holistic approach was working. Blood test after blood test, my PSA continued to drop. On September 24, 2008, my PSA was 0.45. My doctor was so impressed that he requested a copy of my holistic formula and asked me to give a talk at his next patient conference. He also referred me to a prominent doctor at the University of Michigan who specialized in alternative medicine.

It took twenty-six months for my PSA to decline from 2.39 to 0.45. Due to the fact that my PSA levels dropped slightly after each blood draw, I must conclude that my holistic recipe made the difference.

According to Web MD, there is no cure for advanced prostate cancer, only treatments that drastically alter your quality of life. The National Cancer Society reports the five-year survival rate is 30 percent. None of my doctors even told me that there is no cure. In fact, when I asked my doctor after treatment if I was cured, he had no response.

After living through hell for six months, the horrible treatment only lasted nine months. Almost everyone chooses traditional treatment because that is the only choice the medical community offers. A lot of people said it took courage for me to walk away from it and try something new. However, if everyone researched like I did to see the road they wanted me to travel, it really wasn't courage but logic. The road they wanted me to take led to no quality of life and eventual death. The way I looked at it was to roll the dice, and gamble and hope I would beat the odds. With the help of God, I did it.

Since my approach was holistic and used the body to heal itself, it was a slow process that took over a year to accomplish. However, each test showed improvement, which made me feel good because I knew I was going to win. The thought of dying never entered my mind. That is the power of positive mental imaging.

In 2009, I was motivated to share the knowledge I acquired by writing a book, *Advanced Prostate Cancer and Me: How I Reduced My PSA 100% Holistically*. That book helped many people beat cancer or live longer than if they had not used my approach. The letters and feedback from people all over the world made it worth my time. I invested more time and money than I received, which only illustrates that I was not motivated by greed; otherwise, I wouldn't be writing this book. I have been given this information in order to share it with the world. Like my previous book, I am sure I will be attacked and mocked by those that have monetary stakes. My previous book and I were attacked by the greedy pharmaceuticals. I was naive enough to think that when it came to people's lives, greed would not be part of the equation.

I have been doing my protocol since July 2006, making an adjustment here and there. I have added vitamin D, which we will go into detail about in another chapter as to why this vitamin deserves more attention. Then in July 2011, I added a mushroom extract due to the fact it is supposed to strengthen your immune system in order for it to target the stem cells of the cancer. What drew my interest to it was somebody posted a study about it and the cancer board removed it ASAP.

After doing more research on the mushroom extract, I found out it is used as a traditional cancer treatment in Japan and China. Japan has done a number of clinical trials with this extract, and it increased survivability of prostate, breast, colon and lung cancer patients. I then recruited people that had different stages of cancer to see the effect it had on them and the results were tremendous, which motivated me to do this book.

Chapter Two
Why We are Losing the War on Cancer

According to the National Cancer Society, survivability of all cancers has improved by 2 percent in the last forty years. Now, you can attribute that to earlier diagnosis. For example, forty years ago they didn't have the PSA blood test for prostate cancer; therefore, with earlier diagnosis it improves their survivability statistics because it starts with diagnosis. It also could be a statistical error of margin; in any case, our progression is nonexistent.

To put this in the proper prospective, over the last forty years, we have improved survivability for heart disease by over 60 percent to 80 percent, depending on the study. The public is ignorant of this fact because Big Pharma also controls the media with their advertising power and the propaganda they put out to the news organizations.

The reason their results are awful is that they treat the symptom not the cause. The medical community only treats the tumor; and after they poison, burn and cut it out, they seem amazed why it grows back or spreads to other parts of the body. This occurs for a couple of reasons. Once they shrink, cut or burn the tumor, they have left the stem cell or the root of the cancer alone. This is like cutting your grass and wondering why it grows back—you left the roots alone. That is exactly why the cancer grows back; they left or stimulated the stem cell of the cancer.

According to Dr. Max Wicha, a traditional oncologist at the University of Michigan, the radiation and chemotherapy treatment actually awakens the hibernating stem cell of the cancer seven to eight years later. The treatment is the problem. That is why you see a lot of patients seven to eight years after receiving radiation or chemotherapy have a recurrence and, all too frequently, they are terminal. His complete article is in the appendix.

One of the major problems with cancer is that the symptom is treated, but the cause is ignored. In other words, the cause becomes your responsibility, not the medical community's. In addition, they give you no knowledge on how to fight the cause. If you knew ahead of time that it was your job to treat the cause of the cancer, then you would seek out possible solutions. As far as diet, they tell you to eat a Mediterranean diet or a low-fat diet. Both responses are unacceptable.

The next flaw in their treatment is ignoring your immune system and the power of the body to heal itself. In fact, their treatment actually weakens your immune system. In Germany, Switzerland and Japan, when you get cancer treatment, they give you herbs and supplements along with the chemotherapy, and they use a much lower dose than we do. All of their studies demonstrate that a cancer patient's survivability improves when given special supplements.

Our doctors are not trained in nutrition—my daughter, who is a doctor, was trained a whole two hours on nutrition. Whenever you ask an oncologist what your diet should consist of, they answer in vague or "whatever you like" terms. They don't seem to know how Omega-6 feeds cancer. They almost never mention anything about drinking water, or eating organic foods and grass-fed beef. Again they seem to care less about the cause.

If you ask an oncologist, "Why did I get cancer?" they normally respond that it's because it is in your genes. That only plays a part in it, and it is possible to change your genes. A mushroom extract was able to turn off bad genetic genes in mice, all having prostate cancer, in the Australian study of forty mice programmed to get prostate cancer. Twenty were given turkey tail mushroom extract at birth and throughout their lives. Not one developed prostate cancer! On the other hand, the twenty that didn't receive the mushroom extract, each and every one of them, developed prostate cancer. I asked my daughter, the doctor, if is it possible to turn off the switch for bad genes and she concurred that it is possible. So much for the doctor's gene theory that there was nothing you could have done or can do.

The next fallacy is that your diet is not important. I will go into this in great detail in the diet chapter. From my research, Omega-6 needs to be avoided as much as possible. Therefore, you need to eliminate all corn products. Yes, that means you need to read food labels and avoid corn starch, corn fructose, and especially all sodas. You also need to eat and drink organic as much as possible in order to avoid pesticides, herbicides, genetically modified food, growth hormones and antibiotics. As far as milk and meat, limit it—eat organic and grass-fed beef. In addition, your water needs to be filtered to eliminate all the chemicals that are added like fluoride.

The pharmaceuticals are a major part of the problem. They control the Food and Drug Administration (FDA) by paying them huge fees when drugs come to the market. The FDA executives are connected to the pharmaceuticals by past employment. Therefore, you have the foxes guarding the hen house. The pharmaceuticals are only interested in treatments. Cure is not part of their vocabulary.

I recently heard of a new drug for advanced breast cancer where it extends your life on the average of six weeks. You've got to be kidding me. We are not looking for six weeks of extended care; we are looking for at least six years. I remember my doctor commenting one day, "I just gave you four more years." He must have thought I was a politician running for office. I wasn't looking for four more years; I was looking for forty more years. Ideally, they would like to find a chemo drug that you would need for twenty years and it wouldn't kill you like the chemo of today. It is against their financial interest to find a cure. In 2009, 864 clinical trials were conducted on cancer treatments, not one was a cure. This is a trillion dollar industry and the medical cost is 20 percent of our GNP.

Some entity attacked my prior book web sites, sending Trojan horses to my personal computer and to my web server. They also ran phony ads about me and my book. I am unable to run Google ads due to the fact some entity sends me jokes and uses up all my clicks. I wonder which entity would do this—the jokes came from RX emails. My former book is misclassified and buried under medical research. In my wildest dreams, I never would have imagined that greed is more important than life. It just shows how naive I was. In fact, that is why I am not going to hold back any information that might save your life.

Chapter Three
Our Bodies were Designed to Heal Themselves

I firmly believe that God put everything on this Earth to heal us. Our bodies were designed to last way over age 100. In fact, Dr. Gary Null, who has done five years of research on anti-aging and disease in a laboratory setting studying the molecular cell, hoping to figure out why we are aging, believes our bodies were designed to last up to 150 years.

Gary Null received his PhD in Interdisciplinary Studies from Union Institute and University, and is a New York State Certified dietitian-nutritionist. After he completed the laboratory study, Dr. Null then decided to research nutrition by traveling to different countries to study their cultures, their diet and their lifestyle, hoping to shed some light on anti-aging. He did this for five years.

Dr. Null discovered that countries like Italy, where they eat whole foods and fresh foods, have long life expectancies and little disease. When he traveled the country to visit with the people, he saw a better diet, much slower pace and a stress-free type of lifestyle. However, with our diet, coupled with our environment, we short change ourselves. Dr. Null points out that in Italy they eat whole foods, fresh fruit and vegetables, and make the lunch meal a major daily event followed by a siesta time, which is a major reason their life expectancy is greater than ours and their pets live almost twice as long as ours. In fact, in our pet food, they grind up dead dogs that might have died from cancer; therefore, we are feeding our pets contaminated food. That is why you should feed your pets organic food.

During Dr. Null's mice experiments, he attempted many ways of treating mice that were programmed to get cancer, some with great success. One of his great successes was treating terminally ill mice, after they were treated with chemotherapy or radiation, with nutrients and diet; and giving them chlorophyll as their only liquid. He was able to extend their lives for a couple years. When he put the mice on the diet recommended by the doctors (the Mediterranean diet), the mice only lived three months—the worst result of all his experiments.

Dr. Null also had Jewish rabbis pray for terminally ill mice and their tumors disappeared; which means that the belief of prayer is not important, the fact is that someone praying for the mice generated positive energy. We have energy all around us—we need to utilize this energy in healing us. In this country we never teach touch healing, whereas in Europe they utilize that practice. Dr. Null was also able to demonstrate positive energy healing with mice as well as Dr. William Bengston experienced. Proving that we are not just body, we are mind and spirit.

Therefore, in order to start healing our bodies, we need to address all the elements involved. Again, we are composed of mind, body and spirit. Yes, you need to fix your body, but you must also fix your mind and spirit if you are going to beat this.

The mind is a powerful healing instrument that needs to be incorporated into your healing plan. So, you must strive to keep a positive mental attitude. Also, if you don't believe in God, you better find him or at least a belief in a greater being, because your spirit is also a very powerful tool. It is okay to ask for God's help. Without it, I would be deceased.

The next thing is to examine your lifestyle. If you are a heavy alcohol drinker or smoker, you must stop immediately in order for your body to start healing itself. Another item to be addressed is exercise. If you do not currently have an exercise routine, you should consult with your physician or health care provider to find out what workout regimen and level of exertion is right for you.

As far as diet, it is critical that you change it to an anti-inflammatory diet, which we'll discuss in more detail later. But, for now, it's important to remember to ask yourself before you eat anything, "Is this going to help kill my cancer or grow it." Some of the worst beverages are soda pop. They contain corn syrup, artificial flavoring, sugar and carbonation. I used to ask women who had breast cancer if they drank soda pop and they all acknowledged that they did. I'm aware this is not a scientific study; however, I found it quite alarming that everyone I asked said that soda was an important part of their diet. Another important food group to stay away from is processed foods. Our bodies were not made to digest these artificial foods, and this is what grows the cancer.

Our immune system is critical in the process to heal and protect us from disease and aging. One of the biggest cover-ups is how 75 percent of our population is deficient in vitamin D, according to some experts. In fact, one study I read stated that if everyone took supplements for vitamin D, the number of cancers would reduce 75 percent.

According to The University Copenhagen micro biology department, without adequate levels of vitamin D your immune system is unable to activate. Vitamin D is more of a hormone than a vitamin. In other words, your body's defense army is sleeping on the job. Vitamin D turns the switch on for your immune system to activate. Most doctors think 30 ng/ml is adequate. Myself, I like to be above 50 ng/ml. Currently, I am at 65 ng/ml.

From all my research, you need at least 4,000 IU a day of vitamin D. A very well-balanced meal will get you 1,250 IU of D daily. The rest you are supposed to get from the sun. However, unless you live in a year-round warm climate near the equator, it is almost impossible to receive it daily. That is why incidence of cancer becomes greater as you move away from the equator. Therefore, you need to take vitamin D supplements. Most doctors will tell you to take 1,000 or 2,000 IU of D$_3$. Personally, I average about 6,000 IU of Vitamin D$_3$ of supplements daily.

We'll discuss vitamin D in more detail, as well as other vitamins and supplements, including food, that will help turn on your immune system, build your immune system and provide nutrients that your body requires to heal itself in the next two chapters. In other words, give it a swift kick in the ass.

As I said before, our bodies were made to heal themselves. God put everything we need on this Earth. However, due to the fact our food supply is filled with Omega-6 and chemicals, and our environment if full of toxins, we need to take supplements in order to give our body the proper nutrients and vitamins it needs to heal itself. We must also nurture and care for it—mind, body and spirit.

I have been researching and searching for just the right combination of diet, herbs, vitamins and supplements required to help the body heal itself. I can humbly say, "I think I've got it."

Chapter Four
You Are What You Eat and Drink

There are foods that are anti-cancer and there are foods that grow your cancer. What you choose to eat is critical. You want to choose a diet that is anti-inflammatory, whole foods and limit your Omega-6. Omega-6 is found in meat fat, corn oil, peanut oil and almost all products that have the word corn in it, like fructose and corn starch.

You also want to stay away from processed meats and food, and non-organic fruit and vegetables as much as possible. The reason is our bodies were not designed to tolerate pesticides, herbicides and genetically modified foods. Therefore, our immune systems spend way too much time dealing with these foreign poisons, thus, allowing cancer to grow and spread.

The reason cancer is on the rise is a direct correlation to our food supply. The fast-food industry now dictates how we manufacture meat, chicken and vegetables. Speed and cost are the primary reasons our food supply is the enemy, health and disease take a backseat. A great movie to watch is *Food Inc.* It depicts where our food industry is and how it got there. I caution you regarding the movie; it might turn you into a vegetarian.

Another issue is what you drink. All soda pops contain corn fructose, carbonation, artificial coloring and chemicals, and are pure poison as far as I am concerned. They should have a warning label like cigarettes, "Drinking this will cause cancer." One study stated that if you drink two sodas a week, you increase the probability of pancreatic cancer 86 percent.

As far as our water, which is filled with chemicals like fluoride and others, I suggest you filter it or order glass purified water. The reason I said glass is all these plastic containers of filtered water may be doing more harm than good. According to my holistic doctor, these plastic containers are transported in non-air-conditioned trucks. In the summer, and in warm climates, some particles of the plastic are melting in the water. Therefore, your immune system is being compromised.

When it comes to alcohol, I suggest you limit your intake to just social drinking or not at all. If you want the grape seed extract, you don't need a glass of wine—you are able to get it without the alcohol. One hour after opening a bottle of red wine, all the health benefits of the grape seed extract are lost.

Another way you can receive nutrients is by using only sea salt. Sea salt contains seventeen nutrients that regular salt does not have. In fact, sea salt is cleaned of the nutrients, and the nutrients are then used to make vitamins. Therefore, I suggest that you use sea salt in order for you to receive these important nutrients.

In regard to sugar, I would limit it as much as possible as we have all read so many articles about how sugar is the enemy. On the other hand, our cells and body require some sugar. Personally, I have not removed sugar from my diet. What I do is merely reduce my intake. However, I do enjoy my candy bars as long as it is dark chocolate, but I stay away from pastries and processed sweets as much as possible. I would also avoid all artificial sweeteners. Our bodies were not designed to digest them; therefore, your immune system must deal with them instead of the cancer.

As far as meat, I limit my intake and choose grass-fed and very lean meat to avoid the Omega-6 that is found in red meat fat. The only milk I drink is organic with DHA Omega-3 in it. Again, I want to avoid the growth hormones and chemicals in regular milk. I truly believe that it was the growth hormones in the milk and meat that advanced my cancer at a young age of fifty-three. By drinking low-fat organic milk with Omega-3 in it, I am simulating the Budwig diet.

The Budwig diet that was discovered by Dr. Johanna Budwig consists of mixing low-fat organic cottage cheese with flaxseed oil, which is rich in Omega-3. She discovered by mixing sulphureted protein—which is in cottage cheese and most dairy products—with Omega-3, it removes the bad fat surrounding your cells with the good fat. Therefore, your cells are now receiving the proper signals from the brain. Before this correction, the bad fat cells were not receiving the signals from the brain; therefore, your battery is dead.

According to Dr. Budwig, this protocol worked for all types of cancer and had an 80 percent to 90 percent success rate. She claims the ones that failed were due to chemotherapy or drugs that compromised the immune system and weakened the body. Again, every morning I drink low-fat organic milk with DHA Omega-3 in it. I would Google Dr. Johanna Budwig if you would like to know more about it.

Super Foods to Conquer Cancer

Asparagus contains vitamin D, folic acid and antioxidant glutathione, all thought to play a role in lowering the risk factors for cancer. In fact, I have heard of a raw diet of asparagus actually curing some people.

Walnuts have three components that help combat cancer: Omega-3, antioxidants and components called phytosterols, which have shown to slow cancer growth.

Anti-Cancer Foods

These foods are considered anti-inflammatory. Inflammation stimulates the production of growth factors and free radicals. Inflammation can lead to immune suppression and can increase the production of proteins that stimulate the growth of tumor blood vessels. Inflammation causes the buildup of free radicals, which impairs the destruction of cancer cells.

- Blueberries
- Broccoli
- Cabbage
- Cranberries
- Dark Chocolate
- Garlic
- Grapes
- Green Tea (Japanese varieties contain the greatest amount of the anticancer phytonutrients)
- Omega-3 fatty acids
- Onions
- Strawberries
- Turmeric

Super Fruits

These fruits are antioxidant and anti-inflammatory. Causes of inflammation are smoking, excessive alcohol consumption, sleep deficit, pollutants, obesity, stress, negative energy, unhealthy dietary fats, unhealthy carbohydrates and unhealthy cooking methods such as deep frying, and high heat methods or charcoal grilling.

- Acai Berries – weapons-grade antioxidant support
- Apples – fiber source, antioxidants that are antihistamine and anti-inflammatory
- Bananas – high in potassium
- Blackberries – antioxidant powers

- Blackberries – in the top ten of antioxidant support
- Blueberries – helps your brain function and memory
- Cantaloupes – vitamin A and good for your skin, your largest organ
- Cherries – antioxidant support called anthocyanin
- Cranberries – prevents urinary-tract infections and ovarian cancer
- Grapes – filled with antioxidant support called Resveratrol
- Kiwi – greatly helps the digestive system
- Lemons – high in vitamin C; I have also heard how it helped a colon cancer patient defeat it
- Oranges – packed with vitamin C, vitamin B, keeps the immune system humming
- Papayas – packed with vitamin C
- Pomegranates – the highest antioxidant support of all foods
- Raspberries – filled with fiber, vitamin C and magnesium
- Strawberries – packed with vitamin C
- Tomatoes – packed with lycopene
- Watermelon – packed with lycopene

Foods to AVOID

Again, I want to list all the bad foods and beverages you need to avoid. You really need to limit your milk and meat intake. Anything that would be considered inflammatory needs to be limited and avoided. Instead of soda pop, I drink tart cherry juice twice a day. Not only does it help in dealing with my cancer but it is also very therapeutic for my arthritis, caused by downhill ski injuries.

- Alcoholic Beverages
- Artificial Sweeteners
- Non-Organic Milk and Meat
- Non-Organic Fruits and Vegetables
- Processed Meats
- Processed Pastries
- Products Containing Corn
- Soda Pop
- Too Much Sugar
- Unfiltered Drinking Water

Seventy percent of all food in the supermarket has Omega-6 in it, disguised as corn starch, corn fructose. Remember, all corn products are bad for us. That is why when I go grocery shopping I stay on the outside aisles. I buy whole foods, organic fruits and vegetables, and organic meat and milk.

When I eat something, I say to myself subconsciously, "Is this going to grow my cancer or kill my cancer." I usually follow my advice approximately 90 percent of the time. I find it almost impossible to follow this all the time. When I go out to eat, I don't follow my advice at all. I will eat non-organic meat, have a beer or two, and throw my diet out the window.

Chapter Five

Holistic Recipes for
Breast, Colon, Lung and Prostate Cancers

My holistic approach is a result of seven years of research and getting very lucky or, for those who do believe in God, divine intervention. Someone is looking out for me. My holistic approach consists with this four-step protocol.

First, detoxify your body to rid yourself of free radicals with Flor Essence tea from the Flora Company in Canada. They are the originators, but there are many copycats out there. I use the eight herb blend.

Second, take supplements to turn on your immune system, to build your immune system and to provide nutrients that your body requires to defeat cancer. The supplements are anti-aging, too.

Third, change your diet to an anti-inflammatory one—eliminate or reduce Omega-6.

Last, start mediating and believing you are going to win. We are energy! Surround yourself with positive people in your support group that includes your doctors. If your doctors are not in favor of your alternative method, terminate them before their negative energy terminates you.

The mind is a powerful instrument that has healing capabilities. One night I was able to sleep twelve uninterrupted hours. I was in a coma state when my tumor reduced 80 percent. I confirmed this the next morning with a diagnostic test. You must remember it is mind, body and soul. You need all three in order to be successful.

I also pray a lot to my God or a higher power. If you don't believe in God, it might be a good time to re-exam your beliefs. Personally, without God, I don't know how I would have survived, especially when it was God who was instrumental in giving me the formula.

Even though I defeated advanced prostate cancer, the reason I am writing protocols for breast, colon and lung cancer is that the five primary supplements are effective for all four cancers and most cancers according to the studies. The BRCA2 gene is faulty for both breast cancer in women and prostate cancer for men. You will see that the Super Five Supplements are common for all four protocols.

What I call the Super Five Supplements would combat most cancers. The super five are Lycopom, turkey tail mushroom extract, Flor Essence tea, vitamin D and vitamin C. These super five supplements would work on most cancers because cancer is caused by the breakdown of your immune system. What these five supplements do is detoxify your system, strengthen your immune system and rid your body of free radicals.

Super Five Supplements

Lycopom by New Chapter (pomegranate extract)

Pomegranate extract puts the cancer cells in a suspended state, and pomegranates have the highest ORAC (oxygen radical absorbance capacity) of any other food group. Why is that important? Due to the fact that it rids the body of free radicals and the buildup of free radicals is a major cause of cancer. The cancer cells that are affected by pomegranates are breast, colon, lung and prostate.

I believe the big addition to my holistic approach was Lycopom. Each capsule is equivalent to eating fifteen pomegranates and one tomato. I was taking two per day, which is the equivalent of eating thirty pomegranates and two tomatoes each day. In addition, Lycopom has antioxidant support: 23 mg rosehips, 8 mg turmeric supercritical extract, saffron powder, rosemary and marigold.

According to the maker of this product, New Chapter, cancer cells need to be fed. Lycopom supplements prevent cancer cells from receiving the necessary nutrients. This effectively starves the cancer at the cellular level. It would not be practical to eat thirty pomegranates and two tomatoes every day; therefore, this supplement is worth its weight in gold.

Turkey Tail Mushroom Extract

The turkey tail mushroom extract strengthens the immune system in a way that it goes after the stem cell of the cancer. Why that is so crucial is that the stem cell of the cancer is the one that causes recurrences and the spread of the disease to other organs and to the bones.

Surgery, radiation and chemotherapy are not targeting the stem cell of the cancer. It was recently discovered that each cancer tumor has its own stem cell. As long as all the traditional treatments ignore the stem cell, we will continue with the rotten results of cancer survivability.

Turkey tail mushroom extract is from Fungi Perfecti, LLC, www.fungi.com. It is item number NXTV2; if they are out of the extract, I would order the capsules.

Flor Essence Tea

This remarkable tea, Flor Essence, has a long history of helping cancer patients. It is comprised of eight herbs that gently detoxify your system: burdock root, sheep sorrel herb, slippery elm bark, watercress herb, Turkish rhubarb, kelp, blessed thistle herb and red clover blossom. I would also highly recommend that you use the tea from the Flora Company since they are the originators of the tea, and there are many copycats who use only four herbs.

Flor Essence originated in Canada in the 1920s and was used to help treat cancer patients. The formula was given to a nurse by an Ojibway Indian medicine man that showed her how to turn herbs into a healing beverage. In 2004, a laboratory study at Indiana University-Purdue reported that high doses of Flor Essence slow the growth of prostate cancer cells. The FDA has not approved Flor Essence to treat cancer. I can only state the effect it had on me. I drank it religiously from June 2005 to July 2006, and continue to drink it two months a year for a gentle detoxification.

Vitamin D

As we have already discussed, without adequate levels of vitamin D your immune system is unable to activate, and our immune system is critical in the process of healing and protecting us from disease and aging.

You can safely take up to 10,000 IU of vitamin D daily. The Institute of Medicine (IOC) report that says you only need to take 600 IU of vitamin D is only based on bone health, not your immune system. It is also another corrupt report where people with special interests influenced the report. In addition, the media is telling you to stay out of the sun and, if you must be in the sun, be sure to use sunblock—using skin cancer as a fear tactic for you to deprive yourself of adequate levels of Vitamin D, which causes diabetes, heart disease and cancer, just to name a few of the consequences of deficient vitamin D.

One of the first things you really need to do is test your vitamin D level. A simple blood test can determine whether you are vitamin D deficient. I cannot emphasize enough how critical it is that your vitamin D level is more than adequate. If you think 5,000 IU is a high level of vitamin D, let me put this in the proper perspective. If you sit in the sun for fifteen minutes without sun-block, your body will absorb 25,000 IU of vitamin D.

When I hear doctors telling their patients to take 1,000 or 2,000 IU of vitamin D, I believe they are committing medical malpractice. It really isn't their fault because this is what they are trained to tell their patients. However, all the studies that I've read indicate that the higher the level of vitamin D you take, the better the results.

It is possible that if you take too much vitamin D, it could become toxic. However, you would have to take a tremendous amount to get to that level of vitamin D—over 10,000 IU of D_3. I have also read a study that states that the ingredients in sunblock have cancer-causing agents. Any time you put a chemical on your skin it is absorbed by your bloodstream. The skin is our biggest organ and the pores absorb the cream directly into the bloodstream.

Vitamin C

Vitamin C is one of the safest and most effective nutrients for protection against immune system deficiencies; therefore, it is critical for a strong immune system. Since vitamin C is water based, we don't retain any excess. All excess is expelled through our urinary system.

Most of us do not consume enough fruit and vegetables; therefore, we become deficient in C. We are supposed to have nine servings of fruit and vegetables a day in order to get the needed vitamin C that the body requires.

Vitamin C has also shown to strengthen weakened immune systems caused by stress, which we all experience in today's fast-paced society. In addition, vitamin C is one of many antioxidants that can protect against damage caused by harmful molecules called free radicals, as well as toxic chemicals and pollutants like cigarette smoke. Free radicals can build up and contribute to the development of health conditions such as cancer, heart disease and arthritis.

Holistic Recipes

My holistic recipes for breast, colon, lung and prostate cancer are on the following pages. Each recipe is specific to the type of cancer.

Remember, these recipes are only one step in the four-step protocol. The first step is to detoxify your body with Flor Essence tea. After a couple of months, you can take breaks from it and do it maybe one month a quarter. As you improve, you should do it at least twice a year for a gentle detoxification.

The last two steps are changing your diet to an anti-inflammatory one, and mediating and believing you are going to win.

Breast Cancer Holistic Recipe

Supplement	Quantity	When to Take
Lycopom by New Chapter	2 capsules	Lunch or Dinner
Turkey Tail Mushroom Extract	15 to 30 drops twice a day	AM and PM
Flor Essence Tea from the Flora Co.	2 ounces twice a day	AM and PM
Selenium	200 MCG	AM
Folic acid	400 MCG	Lunch
Vitamin B_6	100 MG	Lunch
Tart Cherry Juice	8 ounces	Lunch or Dinner
Vitamin D	5,000 IU of D_3	Breakfast
Vitamin E	400 IU	Breakfast
Avemar – Wheat germ extract	500 MG	Once a day
Vitamin C	1,000 MG	Lunch or Dinner
Ginger Root	500 MG	Lunch or Dinner
CO Q10	100 to 200 MG	Breakfast

Breast Cancer Holistic Recipe Notes

Studies have shown that the ETs, or ellagitannin compounds, derived from pomegranate extract can reduce estrogen receptors by inhibiting aromatase activity. In clinical trials in Japan, turkey tail mushroom extract has shown to improve survivability in breast cancer patients. In fact, in Japan, turkey tail mushroom extract is considered a traditional treatment for cancer.

Avemar has shown in numerous studies a reduction of reoccurrence of breast cancer. I have enclosed the studies in the appendix regarding pomegranates, turkey tail mushroom extract and Avemar.

Colon Cancer Holistic Recipe

Supplement	Quantity	When to Take
Lycopom by New Chapter	2 capsules	Lunch or Dinner
Turkey Tail Mushroom Extract	15 to 30 drops twice a day	AM and PM
Flor Essence Tea from the Flora Co.	2 ounces twice a day	AM and PM
Selenium	200 MCG	AM
Folic acid	400 MCG	Lunch
Vitamin B_6	100 MG	Lunch
Vitamin D	5,000 IU of D_3	Breakfast
Vitamin E	400 IU	Breakfast
Vitamin C	1,000 MG	Lunch or Dinner
Ginger Root	500 MG	Lunch or Dinner
CO Q10	100 or 200 MG	Breakfast

As I stated before, pomegranates and turkey tail mushroom extract are effective for colon cancer as the studies in the appendix illustrate, and the Flor Essence tea is important as a gentle detoxification.

Lung Cancer Holistic Recipe

Supplement	Quantity	When to Take
Lycopom by New Chapter	2 capsules	Lunch or Dinner
Turkey Tail Mushroom Extract	15 to 30 drops twice a day	AM and PM
Flor Essence Tea from the Flora Co.	2 ounces twice a day	AM and PM
Selenium	200 MCG	AM
Folic acid	400 MCG	Lunch
Vitamin B$_6$	100 MG	Lunch
Vitamin D	5,000 IU of D$_3$	Breakfast
Vitamin E	400 IU	Breakfast
Vitamin C	1,000 MG	Lunch or Dinner
Budwig Diet	See Chapter 4	Breakfast
CO Q10	100 or 200 MG	Breakfast

For lung cancer, the Budwig diet is suggested. However, the Budwig diet is good for all four cancers. As always, vitamin D is critical in initiating the immune system.

Prostate Cancer Holistic Recipe

Supplement	Quantity	When to Take
Lycopom by New Chapter	2 capsules	Lunch or Dinner
Turkey Tail Mushroom Extract	15 to 30 drops twice a day	AM and PM
Flor Essence Tea from the Flora Co.	2 ounces twice a day	AM and PM
Selenium	200 MCG	AM
Folic acid	400 MCG	Lunch
Vitamin B_6	100 MG	Lunch
Tart Cherry Juice	8 ounces	Lunch or Dinner
Vitamin D	5,000 IU of D_3	Breakfast
Vitamin E	400 IU	Breakfast
Saw Palmetto Berries	550 MG	Lunch
Vitamin C	1,000 MG	Lunch or Dinner
Ginger Root	500 MG	Lunch or Dinner
CO Q10	100 to 200 MG	Breakfast

Prostate Cancer Holistic Recipe Notes

According to New Chapter, what feeds prostate cancer is 5-lipoxygenase (or 5-LO for short). It has been shown to be associated with the production of a chemical called 5-HETE, without which cancer cells in the prostate cannot survive. Simply put, 5-HETE is the only food that cancer cells eat—it is the essential carrot for the malignant rabbits that want to run wildly throughout your body.

What can be done to prevent the body's creation of 5-HETE is to eliminate an enzyme 5-LO, an Omega-6 fatty acid, which is found in red meats, and certain cooking oils like peanut and corn oils. On consumption, ellagitannins (ETs) antioxidants breakdown to metabolites known as urolithins, which inhibit the growth of prostate cancer cells. This is from a study by the American Chemical Society, dated September 25, 2007.

You might also want to add some more B vitamins for more energy, like B_1 and B_{12}.

Chapter Six

How to Boost My Approach for Late-Stage Cancer

In order to boost my approach, I would increase the Lycopom to three a day for stage 3 cancer, and four a day for stage 4 cancer. Pomegranates have the highest antioxidants of all foods. What it does is rid your body of free radicals, which also slows your aging process. Therefore, there isn't a better food that you can take to strengthen your immune system.

The next thing I would do is replace the 1,000 mg of vitamin C with homemade liposomal C. The reason I would do this is that vitamin C is coated and, therefore, it is not absorbed by your digestive system but absorbed by your tissues; thereby, making liposomal C more powerful. In fact, I have read that it is actually more powerful than IV vitamin C. In order to make this homemade vitamin C, you will need a quart jar, an ultrasonic jewelry cleaner and two six-ounce jars with tops.

Homemade Liposomal C Recipe

Step 1: Pour one cup of distilled water into a quart jar. Add three level tablespoons of grandeur soy lecithin then pour it into the sonic jewelry cleaner and agitate vigorously for five minutes. Pour it back into the jar and place the lecithin mixture in the refrigerator for two hours or more. You can leave it in the refrigerator overnight if you prefer. This allows the lecithin granules to soak up water for easy mixing. After two hours of soaking, vigorously agitate the mixture for another three to five minutes. At the conclusion, there should be no granules visible. Set this smooth lecithin mixture aside.

Step 2: Dissolve one level tablespoon of pharmaceutical grade vitamin C powder into two ounces of distilled water. We recommend you use a six-ounce or larger screw-lid jar so you can shake it vigorously.

Step 3: Dissolve a heaping tablespoon of bicarbonate soda into two ounces of distilled water using a separate six-ounce or larger screw-lid jar. Shake or agitate the mixture three minutes or until the soda is dissolved.

Step 4: Pour the lecithin solution into the jewelry cleaner with the vitamin C and bicarbonate of soda mixture, and stir the contents together.

Step 5: Turn the ultrasonic cleaner on and, using a plastic straw, gently, slowly stir the contents. You can raise the level of encapsulation by continuing several more ultrasonic cycles if desired. I personally recommend at least six minutes.

This protocol makes a total of 12 grams of vitamin C, which will give you 70 percent to 90 percent of encapsulation or the equivalent of 8,400 mg. Drink three to four ounces of your homemade liposomal C a day, and keep the rest refrigerated.

You may also want to watch this video that explains the procedure: http://www.youtube.com/watch?v=SeU--wadrMY. If you don't wish to go through this process, you can purchase the encapsulated vitamin C online.

In the event you feel sharp pains throughout your body, this is the vitamin C killing the cancer and leaving holes where the cancer was, which causes the sharp pain. This is a sign that the encapsulated vitamin C is working. The pain should subside in a couple of days and then you can go back to the process.

This is one of the best ways to strengthen your immune system. Coupled with the turkey tail mushroom extract, along with the encapsulated vitamin C, your immune system should start kicking in.

In order for your immune system to actually be turned on, you must have adequate levels of vitamin D_3. As we've already discussed, without adequate levels of vitamin D, your immune system will not switch on. Therefore, it is critical that you have adequate levels of vitamin D_3.

I recommend everyone with cancer double the recommended amount of vitamin D. I personally take 5,000 IU a day. You also need to monitor your D level because if it is over 100 ng/ml, it can become toxic. However, you can safely take up to 10,000 IU of D_3 a day.

In summary, the most important things you can take for your immune system is encapsulated vitamin C, vitamin D, turkey tail mushroom extract and pomegranate extract. If you take all four of these, you should have a very strong immune system. Again, the body is made to heal itself.

Chapter Seven
What You Need to do In Order to Win

In order to beat the beast, it is mind, body and soul. Just strengthening your immune system is not enough. Your mind is a very powerful instrument that must be utilized in this process. Whether you meditate or you think positive thoughts, you must believe you're going to beat this disease. When I was diagnosed with advanced prostate cancer, the thought of me ever dying because of this disease never entered my mind. In fact, one evening prior to all the unusual side effects that I had from the hormone therapy, I was able to meditate sleep for twelve hours straight, and my tumor reduced 80 percent in that time. Was that mind over matter? God only knows.

It is also extremely important to surround yourself with positive energy. If your physician is negative, he or she needs to be terminated. If your spouse is negative, you need to convey to your spouse how important and necessary positive energy is for you to accomplish this goal. I was counseling an individual who had stage 4 prostate cancer; it was in his bones. Even though I never met this individual, I sensed from him that he was very negative about beating this. Regretfully, when I called to follow up, he had passed away. After talking with his wife, who was very negative, I realized he did not have his mind working in a positive force. People that don't believe that your mind is just as important as your body may have a hard time beating this disease.

A great book I read is called *The Energy Cure* by William Bengston, PhD. In this book, he describes how with energy he could heal almost any disease. He proves that you don't need to have an actual belief but you have to have the process of touch healing. It just shows you that with the proper energy almost anything is possible.

William Bengston is a professor of sociology at St. Joseph College in New York. In his early twenties he received the hands-on healing for his chronic back pain. A self-proclaimed skeptic, he began a thirty-five-year inquiry that has made him one of today's leading researchers into the mastery and power of energy medicine. He was given a technique from a friend on how to touch heal and he decided to see if he could teach his students how to energy heal.

Dr. Bengston did numerous studies of healing cancer tumors in mice by utilizing his students. He also discovered it wasn't important that there was a belief from the person doing the healing. What was more important was that they followed the actual procedure. He proved that anybody can energy heal. According to Dr. Bengston, some cancers are more difficult than others; for example, he found prostate cancer was more difficult than lung cancer to heal.

Here is the process from Bengston on how to touch heal. According to Bengston, first make a list of at least twenty things that you don't have and would like—objects, honors, physical or psychological desires. For some reason, if you use less than twenty items, it will not work. You can use more than twenty but you can't use less than twenty. Then you must visualize that each of these items have already been granted. You should choose a means to an end. Don't just put down a pile of money; instead, visualize the actual object, like a pearl white Cadillac Seville. You need to make each object personal, completely selfish and equal in importance. Forget about things like world peace or child hunger, etc.

The next thing is you must do something called "cycling." You need to memorize the list and practice cycling the list over and over until it is memorized, then repeat the list over and over again; the faster you go, the more energy you will achieve. You would then place your hands over the area that needed healing. You need to do it for approximately thirty minutes at each session. However, I did try to heal my ex-girlfriend's broken ankle, which had more damage than touch healing could resolve, so she had to have numerous surgeries. When I would cycle, my palms would begin to hurt from the energy that was passing through it. You will know when you've mastered the technique when you find yourself automatically cycling while experiencing an emotion without having to prompt yourself.

The reason this is effective is that you are silencing the brain that does the analyzing and thinking, and allowing your subconscious mind to take over. Normally, the subconscious mind is secondary to the analyzing and thinking portion of the mind. In order to meditate, you need to silence this part of your mind and allow the subconscious mind to be the dominant one. According to Bengston, belief in the system is unimportant. He was able to prove it with his mice experiments. Again, if you want to know more about it, you need to purchase his book.

Another belief you must have is a belief in God or a higher power. In other words, you must have some form of spirituality other than yourself. I believe that prayer is paramount. If you don't believe in God, you'd better find him fast. Remember it is mind, body and spirit. You need all three components in order to beat this disease. If we were just the body without a mind or soul, then I would say you don't need the other two. However, we are not just a body, we have a soul. I attempt on a daily basis to meditate at least ten to fifteen minutes a day and I recommend that you do the same. That covers the mind. I also highly recommend that you pray at least ten to fifteen minutes a day. In the event you're an atheist, I would find something to pray to whether it's the sun, the moon or the universe.

Another point I have to address is exercise. It is critical that you do some form of exercise at least three times a week in order to keep your body running properly. According to a study about women with breast cancer, those that exercise have a 50 percent less chance of a reoccurrence. That is huge to have that difference in a reoccurrence scenario.

I've touched on this before about positive energy having a positive mental attitude. That is why it's so critical that every person in your support group has a positive piece in the puzzle. One bad apple can spoil the bunch, which means if one of your caretakers is not positive about everything, either change their attitude or replace them. If your physician is not buying in or positive about what you are doing in order to beat this beast, you need to terminate your physician and find one that will be positive.

A human body has energy and that is why it is so important to have positive energy surrounding your body. I know you are thinking, "How can I be positive when I have this rotten stinking cancer?" You have to remember you caused the cancer because of your diet, lifestyle and/or genetics. You can change your diet and lifestyle, and you can turn off the switches of your bad genes. Therefore, you have to look at this as a challenge and a task. After defeating this beast, you come out the other side a much better person.

Another point is you must do your research and get multiple opinions. Do not allow one so-called expert dictate your future. When I was in my research stage, I consulted with six physicians and did my own research. I looked at these physicians as though they were on my board of directors and I was the chairman of the board. I would ask each physician their opinion, then I would do my own research; and based on what I figured out, I would make the final decision.

Too many patients give their doctors a god complex, and will do whatever they tell them to do. People, like my parents, never asked for a second opinion. Due to that, my father was misdiagnosed, which led to his death at a premature age. My parents were from the old school, "Whatever the doctor says, that's what I will do." If I did that, I would be dead today. In addition to that, some people's philosophy is, "If my doctor didn't tell me to do it, I'm not going to do it." I can't help those people. As you know, my daughter is a physician, and her opinion counted; however, there were many times I went against her advice.

It is important to remember that it is your body, not the doctor's, and doctors are humans, not gods. All the studies show that those patients that used supplements in addition to traditional treatment had much better survivability than those that didn't. I remember my doctor telling me not to use supplements as it would grow the cancer. I then requested that he put me in the direction of any studies that indicate what he just said; of course, he couldn't. Another good point is the doctor works for you, you don't work for the doctor; you're the employer, he or she is the employee. However, too many people are intimidated by doctors and, therefore, do whatever they say. In fact, I knew of an individual who was diagnosed the same month I was—same cancer, same stage, same treatment, same date of recurrence. He decided to go through the traditional hormone treatment and only followed his doctor's advice. Regrettably, he died January 2009, almost four years after diagnosis.

The sole purpose of this book is to be a manual on how to beat cancer. This is not an à la carte menu where you pick and choose which steps you want to take. It's very important that you do all the steps, and you really need to cut or eliminate Omega-6 from your diet.

When it comes to the actual recipes of my protocol, I would strongly suggest that you choose all, not just the Lycopom, Vitamin D and encapsulated Vitamin C. They all work together and they're all needed. As far as the Flor Essence tea, you don't need to do it all the time. I would do the tea for two or three months, and then maybe one month a quarter. As you improve, you should do it at least one month every six months.

I also highly recommend that you check your vitamin D level with a simple blood test. You should know what is going on with your D Level. As far as the averages of vitamin D, I suggest that you don't use the 30 ng/ml measurement as normal. As a cancer patient, you need a number of 50 or above, not to exceed 100.

Afterword

As I look back on my situation—getting cancer at a young age of fifty-three—I realize something very good came out of this. I am now able, with what I've learned, to help many people all around the world. The main reason I'm writing this book is to help people. I am also sick of hearing that there was nothing that could have been done for him or her. I feel I was very fortunate to have found everything I needed to beat this beast. I believe the reason I was given this information was to share it with the world. I don't want to leave this Earth knowing that I did not do everything I was supposed to do. I believe this is the purpose of my life.

All of my information has come to me by mysterious ways, such as how I found my holistic medical doctor or, in a way, how he found me. I had not considered going to a holistic doctor; however, a business associate suggested it. His brother-in-law just happened to be one. He had to pull strings to get me in right away. Normally there was at least a three-month wait for new patients. Also, how my girlfriend came into the picture was also very mysterious. She came up North looking for me at a ski resort after my treatment. She had met me previously and I must have had an impact on her. The reason I am explaining all this is because I am just the messenger. I never asked for this, but everything that has evolved and how information gravitates towards me has me thinking this is not just a coincidence, it is destiny.

I do not have a medical background and I majored in business in college. I had a traumatic event as a child that makes me want to run from doctors and hospitals. When I was nine years old, I spent eleven months in a hospital, not allowed to leave my bed with a bleeding kidney. Today you would be out of the hospital in forty-eight hours. After that experience, I never wanted to see, let alone work in a hospital. My daughter is a physician. Most of my friends growing up are now physicians. However, I believe everything happens for a reason, and if I were a physician, I wouldn't have been allowed to think outside the box and be writing this book on how I cured myself. I believe in using all the tools in the toolbox.

What I did when I was diagnosed was to get multiple opinions and do my own research. I also took notes and wrote my questions prior to meetings with numerous doctors, and I wrote down the answers during the meetings. I learned at a young age that not all doctors are good, and by no means are they a god. After researching all the treatments, I chose a procedure that would give me the best chance of a quality life and was most logical with my situation. Therefore, I chose external beam radiation with short-form hormone treatment. I never understood why they called it hormone a treatment when, in fact, it is really chemical castration. Hormone treatment stops the production of testosterone, which will cause all sorts of problems.

You probably noticed that I never discussed pH levels. There are too many books already on it. If you control the pH level, you kill your cancer. I am in partial agreement about their philosophy, but it's too simplistic to think that you don't need body, mind and soul. The books about pH only discuss the body, which is only one third of the equation. I truly believe that if you don't incorporate the soul and your spiritual self, you'll have a difficult time. I am also a strong believer in positive mental energy. The mind is a powerful tool that you must incorporate one way or the other. It's amazing that if your mind can perceive it, you can see it happening.

I don't care who I offend or which groups feel that I've hurt them. If some of those groups really cared about saving people's lives, they would incorporate some of my ideas. However, it's all about greed with them. You're probably wondering which group I'm talking about. It happens to be the pharmaceutical industry. They believe if it is not a drug that they can profit from, they are against it. One example is that the Institute of Medicine (IOM) has just come out with a statement saying that no one should take any form of vitamin D supplements. In their previous reports they recommended only 600 IU of vitamin D, knowing that it is very inadequate and will lead them to huge profits.

As stated before, I read a study that said if everybody had sufficient levels of vitamin D, all diseases, including cancer, would reduce by 75 percent. That is huge. That is why Big Pharma puts out these phony reports. I also read another study on Web MD regarding pregnant women taking vitamin D supplements. They broke up each group with different levels of vitamin D up to a maximum level of 4,000 IU a day. The group that took the 4,000 IU a day had the healthiest babies and the easiest deliveries. At the time, taking 4,000 IU of D was considered risky, and they were concerned it would be too much and had that group sign waivers. I cannot emphasize enough the importance of vitamin D.

The entire way they treat cancer, which is treating the symptom not the cause, is totally backwards. Cancer is caused by the breakdown of your immune system. Therefore, it makes perfect sense to strengthen and repair your immune system. Let the body heal itself.

It is almost comical to hear the medical community say, "Oh well, we shrunk the tumor 30 percent." Until they deal with the stem cell of the cancer, they will never make any real progress. I like to use this analogy: The way they treat cancer is the way they cut grass. They get rid of what they can see, but they leave the roots to grow back. That is why the reoccurrence and the survival rate are so poor for most cancers. In fact, a well-known leading oncologist at the University of Michigan, Max Wicha, believes what we need is a treatment that targets the stem cell of the cancer. He goes on to say that radiation and chemotherapy stimulate the hibernating stem cells to come back approximately seven years after treatment. That is what causes a reoccurrence for these individuals.

To me, the definition of insanity is doing the same thing and expecting different outcomes. That is how cancer is treated. They use the same failed procedures over and over again, and the public is completely ignorant of this fact. If my cancer ever comes back, I will never consider traditional treatment. It is barbaric and backwards. They treat the symptom, not the cause. You can't cut, burn and poison cancer and expect no recurrence, especially when you ignore the stem cell. We need to deal with the cause and the symptom. Until we deal with it logically, we will never get anywhere with cancer.

For further updates, questions, testimonials and comments, please visit my web site at www.ibeatcancerholistically.com. I hope and pray that this book saves and extend many lives. God bless you all.

Appendix
Research Articles

Pomegranate Compounds Inhibit Aromatase and Reduces Breast Cancer Cell Proliferation

Posted: January 5, 2010

Published by: Food for Breast Cancer, http://foodforbreastcancer.com/news/pomegranate-compounds-inhibit-aromatase-and-reduces-breast-cancer-cell-proliferation
News type: Breast cancer study
Publication: Cancer Prevention Research, January 2010
Study name: Pomegranate Ellagitannin-Derived Compounds Exhibit Antiproliferative and Antiaromatase Activity in Breast Cancer Cells In vitro

A new study has demonstrated that ellagitannin compounds derived from pomegranate fruit can reduce estrogen receptor positive (ER+) breast cancer proliferation by inhibiting aromatase activity. Estrogen stimulates the growth of ER+ tumors. Androgen is converted to estrogen in the body by the aromatase enzyme, thereby promoting such breast cancer. Pomegranate fruit, which is a rich source of ellagitannins, has attracted notice because of its reported anticancer and anti-atherosclerotic properties. Pomegranate ellagitannins hydrolyze upon consumption, releasing ellagic acid, which is then converted to various derivative compounds by microflora in the gut. In the study, 10 ellagitannin-derived compounds were tested. All were found to exhibit antiproliferative activity, and six were found to have anti-aromatase activity, the strongest of which was demonstrated by urolithin B. Further testing demonstrated that urolithin B significantly inhibited testosterone-induced MCF-7aro cell proliferation. MCF-7aro breast cancer cells are estrogen receptor positive/aromatase positive and demonstrate increased cell proliferation in the presence of testosterone. The authors conclude that pomegranate ellagitannin-derived compounds have potential for the prevention of estrogen-responsive breast cancers.

Other studies have also reported chemopreventive activities of pomegranates

Previous studies have also found that pomegranate-derived compounds inhibit aromatase in breast cancer cells. Studies have also found other anti-breast cancer activities of pomegranates:

- Punicic acid, a component of pomegranate seed oil, has been found to reduce the growth and proliferation of estrogen-negative (ER-) breast cancer cells
- Delphinidin, a major anthocyanin present in pomegranates and other pigmented fruits and vegetables, has been shown to possess potent antioxidant and antiproliferative properties in HER2 overexpressing breast cancer cells
- Pomegranate seeds contain a large fraction of conjugated linolenic acid, which has been shown to have chemopreventive effects against cancer
- Pomegranate seed oil and fermented pomegranate juice polyphenols have both been shown to inhibit anglogenesis in both ER+ and ER- breast cancer cells
- Pomegranate juice has been found to inhibit proliferation of ER- breast cancer cells in a dose- and time-dependent manner to a degree comparable to that of high-dose Cisplatin chemotherapy
- A pomegranate extract has been found to greatly inhibit tumor growth in Her2/neu transgenic mice
- Pomegranate juice has been found to have greater antiproliferative, apoptotic and antioxidant activities than individual pomegranate components, including punicalagin, ellagic acid, and pomegranate tannins, suggesting that compounds in the juice act synergistically compared to single purified active ingredients

Avemar: The Wheatgerm Extract That May Help Reduce Cancer Reoccurrence

Date: 05/05/06

Published by: The Healthier Life,
http://www.thehealthierlife.co.uk/natural-health-
articles/cancer/avemar-wheatgerm-extract-reduce-cancer-
reoccurrence-00104.html

Since 1996, over 100 studies done on Avemar have impressed oncologists and cancer researchers. Studies have shown that when Avemar is used as an adjunct treatment, it enhances the effects of the standard treatment agents. Its particularly effective in reducing the chances of cancer reoccurrence...

Cancer treatment has come a long way since the use of mustard gas derivatives in the early 1900s or has it? When doctors discovered during World War I that mustard gas destroyed bone marrow, they began to experiment with it as a way to kill cancer cells. Although they had little success with the mustard gas, it did pave the way for modern chemotherapy which involves the most toxic and poisonous substances anyone deliberately puts in his body. These treatments kill much more than cancer cells they have a devastating effect even on healthy ones.

Sometimes it seems as if only a miracle could provide a cure thats both safe and effective. And a miracle is just what Dr. Mate Hidvegi believed he found when he patented Avemar. Studies have shown that Avemar, a fermented wheatgerm extract, helps reduce cancer reoccurrence, possibly speed up cancer cell death and helps the immune system identify cancer cells for attack.

A miracle in the making

Back in World War I, Dr. Albert Szent-Gyrgyi (a Nobel Prize recipient in 1937 for his discovery of vitamin C) had seen the effects of mustard gas personally and was determined to find a safer alternative for cancer treatment. His goal was to prevent the rapid reproduction that is characteristic of cancer cells. He theorised that supplemental quantities of naturally occurring compounds in wheatgerm called DMBQ would help to chaperone cellular metabolism, allowing healthy cells to follow a normal course but prohibiting potentially cancerous ones from growing and spreading. His early experiments, published in the 1960s, confirmed his theory.

But then the science community shifted its focus to killing cancer outright. It wasnt until the fall of communism in Hungary in 1989 when scientists were allowed for the first time to pursue independent, personal interests that Dr. Hidvegi picked up where Szent-Gyrgyi left off.

He was able to patent a technique of fermenting wheat germ with bakers yeast. He named this fermented product Avemar and it became the standard compound for research and later commercialisation because it assured a longer shelf life while maintaining its live food status.

Reduce cancer reoccurrence

Since 1996, over 100 studies done on Avemar have impressed oncologists and cancer researchers. Studies have shown that when Avemar is used as an adjunct treatment, it enhances the effects of the standard treatment agents. Its particularly effective in reducing the chances of cancer reoccurrence.

In a controlled study, 170 subjects with primary colorectal cancer either had surgery and standard care with chemotherapy or the same plus 9g of Avemar taken once a day. Only 3 per cent of the people in the Avemar group experienced a reoccurrence, vs. more than 17 per cent of those in the chemo-only group. The Avemar group also showed a 67 per cent reduction in metastasis and a 62 per cent reduction in deaths.

In a randomized study, 46 stage III melanoma patients with a high risk of reoccurrence either had surgery and standard care with chemotherapy or surgery plus standard care and 9g of Avemar taken once a day. Those taking Avemar showed approximately a 50 per cent reduction in risk of progression.

Avemar also reduced the frequency and severity of many common side-effects, including nausea, fatigue, weight loss and immune suppression.

Avemar speeds cancer cell death

The second way Avemar works against cancer is to help keep cancer cells from repairing themselves. Cancer cells reproduce quickly and chaotically, producing many breaks and other mistakes in the cellular structure. Because of this, cancer cells need a lot of the enzyme known as PARP (poly-ADP-ribose) to help repair breaks in DNA before the cells divide. It is thought that without adequate PARP, cancer cells cannot complete DNA replication. When theres no PARP to repair the damage, an enzyme called Caspase-3 initiates programmed cell death.

Avemar has been shown to potentially speed up the death of cancer cells by helping inhibit the production of PARP and enhancing the production of Caspase-3.

US researchers at UCLA also showed that Avemar may reduce the production of RNA (ribonucleic acid) and DNA associated with the rapid reproduction of cancer cells. It also helps restore normal pathways of cell metabolism and may increase the production of RNA and DNA associated with healthy cells.

Undercover cancer cells exposed

Avemar may also act as a biological bounty hunter for hidden cancer cells. Healthy cells have a surface molecule called MHC-1 that tells natural killer (NK) cells not to attack. Virally infected cells dont display this molecule, which makes them targets.

However, cancer cells have also been shown to display the surface molecule MHC-1, which means that cancer cells may actually be able to hide from NK cells. Avemar is thought to help the immune system identify cancer cells for attack by suppressing their ability to generate this MHC-1 mask, which allows the NK cells to recognize it as a target for attack.

What to take for best results

The Avemar product is an instant drink mix called Av, which combines Avemar with natural orange flavouring and fructose in pre-measured packets. As a dietary supplement, the recommended usage is one packet per day mixed with 8oz of cold water.

You should consume it within 30 minutes of mixing a batch. Also note that its a good idea to take Av one hour before or after a meal and two hours before or after any drugs or other dietary supplements. If you weigh over 200 pounds (14 stone), use two packets per day. If you weigh less than 100 pounds (7 stone), only use half of a packet per day.

Although some people reported uneasiness in their stomachs during the first few days of using Avemar, the effect only lasted a few days. No vomiting, diarrhoea, or any other symptoms were reported.

Contraindications: Since this is a wheat product, there is the potential for allergic response. Avemar should not be consumed by people who have had an organ or tissue transplant, those who have malabsorption syndrome, or those with allergies to foods containing gluten, such as wheat, rye, oats and barley. Its also not recommended for people with fructose intolerance or hypersensitivity to gluten, wheatgerm, or any of the components or ingredients of this product.

If you suffer from bleeding ulcers, you should stop using Avemar two days before undergoing a barium X-ray contrast examination and resume taking it two days after the completion of the examination. This precaution is necessary because wheatgerm contains lectin, which can potentially cause red blood cells to clump. If you are currently taking medications or have any adverse health conditions, you should consult with your pharmacist or physician before taking Avemar.

Sources:
1. British Journal of Cancer 2003; 89(3): 465-9
2. International Journalof Cancer 2002; 100(S13): 408
3. 'A medical nutriment study has supportive effect in oral cancer' (unpublished, Marta Ujpal et al)
4. Pancreas 2001; 23: 141-7; Drug Discovery Today 2002; 7(6): 18-26
5. Journal of Bilogical Chesmistry 2002; 277: 46,408-14; International Journal of Oncology 2002; 20: 563-70

Turkey Tail Mushroom Extract for Cancer Treatment

Published by: Medicinal Mushrooms, http://medicinal-mushrooms.net/turkey-tail-mushroom-extract-for-cancer-treatment/

Turkey Tail mushrooms are known to be a well-researched and the most revered medicinal fungi all over the world, but particularly in Japan and China. It is a herbal mushroom that has an tremendous amount of health benefits that anyone can imagine. Known in a variety of names, like Coriolus versicolor, Trametes versicolor, Polystictus versicolor, Kawaratake and Yun Zhi, they thrive well in the northern parts of Europe, China and Japan. It can also be seen proliferating in the thick forests of many areas in the United States, Canada and Siberia. The plant is highly regarded in Japan and China because of its effectiveness as a herbal medicine.

Turkey Tail Mushrooms, when eaten raw, are leathery and chewy. This is why most users consume them by making tea out of them. One can make a medicinal beverage out of turkey tail mushroom extracts by boiling them for a long period of time. However, a number of long-time users swear to the mushrooms' optimal effectiveness by chewing them.

Active, medicinal compounds are the reasons why the turkey tail mushroom extract is recognized as one of the leading form of herbal treatment in Japan. In a number of Japanese clinical studies and trials, the mushrooms extended survival rates of people who had breast cancer, lung cancer, cancer of colon-rectum, cancer of the esophagus and prostate cancer. Turkey Tail Mushroom was so successful in exhibiting medicinal properties that it was approved by Japan's Ministry of Health and Welfare, to be used as a significant cancer treatment. Turkey Tail Mushroom, or Trametes versicolor, exhibited not only anti-tumor, but also anti-inflammation and antiviral effects, as well. It also fights serious liver problems, like chronic active hepatitis and hepatitis B.

Medicinal Benefits of Turkey Tail Mushroom

Numerous scientific researches and studies pointed to the fact that Turkey Tail Mushroom extract provides a host of medicinal and health effects on users. These include:

- Immune-stimulating, enhancing and strengthening effects
- Cytotoxic T-cell stimulation and natural killer or NK enhanced cell activity
- Anti-viral effects against human papilloma virus, herpes and Epstein Barr virus
- Anti-bacterial effects
- Anti-cancer effects, like as pro-apoptosis and anti-angiogenic activities
- Anti-tumor effects, like inhibition of tumor cell invasion and migration

Important Source of Polysaccharide-K

Trametes versicolor, as a number of scientists refer to Turkey Tail mushrooms, is obviously significant for a variety of medical reasons. However, they are well-known for being a natural source of polysaccharide PSK, which is an anti-cancer compound. Extensive research has actually identified two polysaccharide-protein components, known as proteoglycan, of Trametes versicolor responsible for these anticancer effects, PSK and Polysaccharide-protein complex, or PSP. However, PSK is far more abundant than PSP, and so, is more utilized for most clinical studies and treatments.

PSK is a high-concentrated molecular weight carbohydrate that is found to exist in abundance in fruit bodies. Furthermore, it is discovered to be present in much higher concentrations in the mycelium part of Turkey Tail mushrooms. There have been studies on extracts from Coliorus versicolor (Turkey Tail), which proved that they can be used positively as a supplementary treatment for radiation therapy and chemotherapy. Indeed, because of the relative abundance of PSK in these Oriental fungi, more and more cancer specialists and immunologists now consider it as a key cancer treatment.

Maintenance of the immune system and liver function

It has been proven by a number of clinical research and studies in Japan and China that the defenses of the body can be strengthened at its most basic level with the 100 percent immunity-protection properties of Turkey Tail Mushroom. Traditional Japanese and Chinese healers have long revered Turkey Tail Mushroom for its valuable parts and extracts. Such ingredients are used to create natural medicinal tonics meant for strengthening the immune system and maintaining a healthy liver function. At the same time, modern medicine has shown that Turkey Tail Mushroom, because of the PSK compounds that it contains, significantly provided strong support to the cellular defenses of the body. Generally, when one uses Turkey Tail Mushroom extract, he is guaranteed at least 25 percent polysaccharide concentration. This guarantees high potency in the strengthening of Immune system and liver function.

PSK targeting cancer stem cells and cancer cell lines

Turkey Tail Mushroom extract has the ability to hinder prostate cancer growth and spread, according to leading trials in Australia. These Australian researches showed that conventional methods of treatments, like radiotherapy and chemotherapy, were able to stop cancerous cells, but not the cancer stem cells. Such cells are that ones that actively initiate the disease and cause it to spread. However, Polysaccharopeptide or PSP, like PSK, effectively targets and destroys prostate cancer stem cells. It also exhibited anti-tumor effects on trials made with mice.

More and more scientists are inclined to believe that cancer stem cell is a key reason why many cancer treatments turn to be futile. With the discovery of Turkey Tail Mushroom extract as highly effective in targeting cancer stem cells, cancer treatments can see some significant success.

Human clinical trials likewise revealed that PSK reduce the recurrence of cancer when utilized as an adjuvant. Similar scientific research has demonstrated that the mushroom is capable of inhibiting some human cancer cell lines. Further studies have shown that PSK, in combination with other medicinal fungal extracts, inhibit proliferation of certain cancer cells.

Major Alternative Medicinal Treatment

It is inevitable that, with the continuous medicinal success of Turkey Tail Mushroom, it is bound to become a vital, significant fixture in the medical field, focusing mainly on the treatment of cancer. A long-time traditional agent in the treatment of cancer cells and boosting of the immune system, it is now being proposed as a possible inhibiting agent of HIV replication. Apart from a being an effective cancer cell killer, Turkey Tail's PSK is now identified to be an efficient agent capable of regenerating sick bone marrow. This is apart from its long-proven capabilities of increasing one's level of energy and providing basic pain relief in patients afflicted with cancer and other serious diseases.

Mushroom Extract Can Stop Prostate Cancer: Study

Updated: 2011-05-25 16:38

Published by: China Daily,
http://europe.chinadaily.com.cn/world/2011-
05/25/content_12583420.htm

CANBERRA - An extract from a mushroom can stop the growth of prostate cancer, Australian researchers said on Wednesday.

According to Patrick Ling from the Australian Prostate Cancer Research Center in Queensland, conventional treatments, like chemotherapy and radiotherapy, targeted some cancer cells, but not stemcells, which initiate cancer and cause the disease to spread.

However, the scientists conducted a study finding that a compound called polysaccharopeptide (PSP), extracted from the turkey tail mushroom, can target prostate cancer stemcells and suppress tumor formation in trials on mice.

"People believe that the cancer stemcell is one of the major reasons why the cancer treatment is not working," he told Australia Associated Press on Wednesday.

"If you can come up with some treatments that can target those cancer stemcells you may actually be able to improve treatments.

"We find that this mushroom extract is very effective in targeting those cancer stemcells."

In a trial involving almost 20 mice carrying a gene to develop prostate cancer, scientists fed PSP to about half for 20 weeks while the others went without.

All of those eating the extract did not develop the cancer, the others did.

Ling said the findings support that PSP may be a potent preventative agent against prostate cancer, through targeting of the prostate cancer stem cell population.

The turkey tail mushroom is used in Asian soups to boost health, but Ling said there is no research to suggest that simply eating the vegetable can have the same effect as his research has found.

More tests will be done later this year.

Vitamin D Crucial to Activating Immune Defenses

Date: 2010-03-07

Published by: University of Copenhagen, http://news.ku.dk/all_news/2010/2010.3/d_vitamin

Scientists from the Department of International Health, Immunology and Microbiology have discovered that Vitamin D is crucial to activating our immune defenses and that without sufficient intake of the vitamin, the killer cells of the immune system - T cells - will not be able to react to and fight off serious, life-threatening infections in the body.

For T cells to detect and kill foreign pathogens such as clumps of bacteria or deadly viruses, the cells must first be 'triggered' into action and 'transform' from inactive and harmless immune cells into killer cells that are primed to seek out and destroy all traces of a foreign pathogen.

The researchers found that the T cells rely on vitamin D in order to activate and they would remain dormant, 'naïve' to the possibility of threat if vitamin D is lacking in the blood.

"We have discovered that the first stage in the activation of a T cell involves vitamin D, explains Professor Carsten Geisler from the Department of International Health, Immunology and Microbiology. When a T cell is exposed to a foreign pathogen, it has an immediate biochemical reaction and extends a signaling device or 'antenna' known as a vitamin D receptor, with which it search for vitamin D. This means that the T cell must have vitamin D or activation of the cell will cease. If the T cells cannot find enough vitamin D in the blood, they won't even begin to mobilise."

T cells that are successfully activated transform into one of two types of immune cell. They either become killer cells that will attack and destroy all cells carrying traces of a foreign pathogen or they become helper cells that assist the immune system in acquiring "memory". The helper cells send messages to the immune system, passing on knowledge about the pathogen so that the immune system can recognize and remember it at their next encounter and launch a more efficient and enhanced immune response. T cells form part of the adaptive immune system, which means that they function by teaching the immune system to recognize and adapt to constantly changing threats.

Activating and Deactivating the Immune System

For the research team, identifying the role of vitamin D in the activation of T cells has been a major breakthrough.

"Scientists have known for a long time that vitamin D is important for calcium absorption and the vitamin has also been implicated in diseases such as cancer and multiple sclerosis, but what we didn't realize is how crucial vitamin D is for actually activating the immune system - which we know now."

The discovery, the scientists believe, provides much needed information about the immune system and will help them regulate the immune response. This is important not only in fighting disease but also in dealing with anti-immune reactions of the body and the rejection of transplanted organs. Active T cells multiply at an explosive rate and can create an inflammatory environment with serious consequences for the body. After organ transplants, e.g. T cells can attack the donor organ as a "foreign invader". In autoimmune disease, hypersensitive T cells mistake fragments of the body's own cells for foreign pathogens, leading to the body launching an attack upon itself.

The research team were also able to track the biochemical sequence of the transformation of an inactive T cell to an active cell, and thus they could intervene at several points to modulate the immune response. Inactive or 'naïve' T cells crucially contain neither the vitamin D receptor nor a specific molecule (PLCgamma1) that would enable the cell to deliver an antigen specific response.

The findings continues Professor Geisler "could help us to combat infectious diseases and global epidemics. They will be of particular use when developing new vaccines, which work precisely on the basis of both training our immune systems to react and suppressing the body's natural defenses in situations where this is important - as is the case with organ transplants and autoimmune disease."

Most Vitamin D is produced as a natural byproduct of the skin's exposure to sunlight. It can also be found in fish liver oil, eggs and fatty fish such as salmon, herring and mackerel or can be taken as a dietary supplement.

Cancer Expert Tells How Treatment Can Be Problem

February 24, 2010
By Mark Roth, Pittsburgh Post-Gazette

Max Wicha is coming to Pittsburgh today to deliver a startling message.

Standard cancer treatments not only often fail to eradicate cancer, but can make it worse.

That argument isn't coming from a fringe proponent of alternative medicine, but from the founder of the University of Michigan's Comprehensive Cancer Center and a pioneer in research on why cancers recur and spread to other parts of the body.

The reason breast cancer and other malignancies often return aggressively after treatment is that when tumor cells die under assault from chemotherapy and radiation, they give off substances that can reactivate a special set of master cells known as cancer stem cells, Dr. Wicha said in an interview Tuesday.

Dr. Wicha's lab has found that inflammatory molecules secreted by dying tumor cells can hook up with the stem cells and cause them in effect to come out of hibernation.

The existence of cancer stem cells is still controversial in some quarters, Dr. Wicha acknowledged, but is gaining traction.

In the last two months alone, researchers around the nation have published studies on cancer stem cells in breast, ovarian, prostate and brain cancer.

Adult stem cells exist in most tissues, and go into action to repair damage from wounds or infections.

In cancer, they can mutate and no longer obey normal bodily signals to stop growing, Dr. Wicha said.

He and other researchers say that even when chemotherapy and radiation cause tumors to shrink dramatically, these stem cells can stay alive, living under the radar until they are once again spurred into action.

They also believe stem cells are probably the ones that break away from an original tumor and cause cancer to spread elsewhere in the body.

Chemo and radiation kill off the fastest-growing cells in the body, which applies to most cancer cells, but the cancer stem cells that create those rapidly dividing tumor cells actually grow much more slowly themselves, and are less susceptible to those therapies, he said.

One tactic to address this problem is to kill off both types of cancer cells at once, Dr. Wicha said.

A recent experimental trial with advanced breast cancer patients at the University of Michigan, Baylor University in Texas and the Dana-Farber Cancer Institute at Harvard University used standard chemotherapy along with a substance designed to block one of the biochemical pathways of stem cells.

The approach killed off more than 90 percent of the cancer stem cells, Dr. Wicha said, and researchers now hope to expand the treatment to a much larger group of patients.

Ultimately, he hopes cancer treatments can avoid general chemo altogether, with its debilitating side effects, and just use targeted therapies against the stem cells.

There is still a long road ahead, he said, and "my feeling is, to really knock these stem cells out, we're probably going to have to use multiple inhibitors."

Vitamin D Deficiency Soars in the U.S., Study Says

New research suggests that most Americans are lacking a crucial vitamin.

By Jordan Lite

Date: March 23, 2009

Published by: Scientific American, http://www.scientificamerican.com/article.cfm?id=vitamin-d-deficiency-united-states

Three-quarters of U.S. teens and adults are deficient in vitamin D, the so-called "sunshine vitamin" whose deficits are increasingly blamed for everything from cancer and heart disease to diabetes, according to new research.

The trend marks a dramatic increase in the amount of vitamin D deficiency in the U.S., according to findings set to be published tomorrow in the *Archives of Internal Medicine*. Between 1988 and 1994, 45 percent of 18,883 people (who were examined as part of the federal government's National Health and Nutrition Examination Survey) had 30 nanograms per milliliter or more of vitamin D, the blood level a growing number of doctors consider sufficient for overall health; a decade later, just 23 percent of 13,369 of those surveyed had at least that amount.

The slide was particularly striking among African Americans: just 3 percent of 3,149 blacks sampled in 2004 were found to have the recommended levels compared with 12 percent of 5,362 sampled two decades ago.

"We were anticipating that there would be some decline in overall vitamin D levels, but the magnitude of the decline in a relatively short time period was surprising," says study co-author Adit Ginde, an assistant professor at the University of Colorado Denver School of Medicine. Lack of vitamin D is linked to rickets (soft, weak bones) in children and thinning bones in the elderly, but scientists also believe it may play a role in heart disease, diabetes and cancer.

"We're just starting to scratch the surface of what the health effects of vitamin D are," Ginde tells *ScientificAmerican.com.* "There's reason to pay attention for sure."

But Mary France Picciano, a senior nutrition scientist in the National Institutes of Health's Office of Dietary Supplements, is skeptical that the dip is as deep or widespread as suggested, noting that there's disagreement on how much vitamin D is needed. She notes that the Institute of Medicine (IOM) defines insufficiency as less than11 nanograms per milliliter. Using that as a threshold, some 10 percent of U.S. adults are vitamin D deficient, according to a study published in November in the *American Journal of Clinical Nutrition.*

That earlier study, co-authored by Picciano, also found that vitamin D deficiency had become more common between the late 1980s and 2004, but that between half and 75 percent of that difference was due to changes in the test used to measure those blood levels and therefore wasn't a true gauge. "The results are far overstated and their findings are not as accurate as ours," Picciano says. "There is some deficiency — I don't want to minimize that — but it's not as high as they're saying."

Ginde insists the results are reliable. "There's potential for methodology contributing to some of what we found," he says, but the magnitude of the change and other research "argue that this is the reality in the U.S. right now."

Ginde, who last month linked vitamin D deficiency to catching more colds, blames increasing use of sunscreen and long sleeves following skin cancer-prevention campaigns for the change. Using a sunscreen with as little as a 15-factor protection cuts the skin's vitamin D production by 99 percent, the study notes, and there are few sources of the vitamin in our diets. Some food sources are salmon, tuna, mackerel and vitamin D-fortified dairy products, such as milk.

IOM recommends that people get 200-600 International Units (IU) of vitamin D daily, but it's reviewing whether to increase that recommendation in the wake of new studies. An update is expected in May 2010. Ginde believes that whatever those recommendations turn out to be, blacks should take double the amount of vitamin D supplements, because they have more melanin or pigment in their skin that makes it harder for the body to absorb and use the sun's ultraviolet rays to synthesize vitamin D. He adds that people should also take greater amounts of vitamin D in the winter when there's less sunlight.

Jim Fleet, a professor of foods and nutrition at Purdue University who wasn't involved in the study, agrees with Picciano that failing to consider differences in the vitamin D testing methods (used during the two survey periods) was "a fatal mistake." But he tells *ScientificAmerican.com* that real deficiencies in vitamin D exist, even when they're defined by the lower cutoff, and that some 40 percent of African Americans are vitamin D deficient according to that threshold.

"If you look at people in the categories that we worry about," he says, "that's still a lot of people."

Institute of Medicine Report on Vitamin D is Wrong, Wrong, Wrong

November 30, 2010

Published by: Alliance for Natural Health, http://www.anh-usa.org/institute-of-medicine-report-on-vitamin-d-is-wrong-wrong-wrong/

A new report, released today by the health arm of the National Academy of Sciences, says that few people are vitamin D deficient. The scientific research says otherwise.

The new Institute of Medicine (IOM) report says that persons between the ages of 1 and 70 do not need more than 600 IU of vitamin D daily—and makes the outrageous claim that few people are actually vitamin D deficient. This is especially troubling considering we're moving rapidly into the thick of flu season, when people need *more* vitamin D, not less.

This is the government's first official vitamin D recommendation since 1997. Despite raising the new vitamin levels by 300% for most Americans, the IOM guidelines are still in contrast to overwhelming scientific evidence that confirms the significant medical benefits of higher vitamin D levels, and that one-third of Americans are vitamin D deficient.

Changes in US lifestyles mean that many people in the US get less exposure to the sun and often inadequate dietary levels of vitamin D. The *New York Times* reports that a number of prominent doctors have advised vitamin D supplementation for a wide variety of illnesses, including heart disease, cancer, and autoimmune diseases. Their research shows that more and more people know their vitamin D levels because they are being tested for it as part of routine physical exams.

The IOM is wrong in its findings, wrong in ignoring the bountiful scientific research that indicates the need for higher levels of vitamin D in our system, and wrong for not educating folks about the ability of vitamin D to combat the flu. Our campaign to end the silence on vitamin D is one attempt to educate the public and get the government to listen to the clear scientific findings.

CPSIA information can be obtained
at www.ICGtesting.com
Printed in the USA
BVOW03s2109011216
469504BV00001B/57/P